From Patient

My Stroke L

By Channa A. G.

Copyright © 2025 by Channa Akurana Gamaralalage.

All rights reserved. No part of this book may be copied, stored, or shared in any form without written permission from the author, except for brief quotations used in reviews or scholarly works.

ISBN: 9798283584508

Printed by Amazon KDP

First Edition – May 2025

Cover design by Channa A. G.

"You don't have to be who you were before the pain. You get to become someone new - someone stronger, wiser, and more alive than ever."

- Channa A. G.

Dedication

*To my beloved wife, **Danushka**,
whose unwavering love, strength, and sacrifice held
me together when I was falling apart.*

*To my son, **Dave**,
whose innocent eyes reminded me every day why I
had to rise again.*

*And to every person facing life's unexpected storms,
May this book be a light in your darkest moment,
a whisper that says, you can begin again.*

Acknowledgement

This book is not just a reflection of my recovery, it is a tribute to the people, experiences, and support that gave me the strength to turn my life around after my stroke.

First and foremost, I would like to thank my wife, Danushka, for being my unwavering support system. Her strength, love, and sacrifices, especially during the times when she had to balance her travel, our family, and my recovery, gave me hope and stability when I needed it most. To my beloved son, Dave, your innocent love and curiosity reminded me daily of why I had to fight harder.

To my medical team at Hull Royal Infirmary, England, thank you for your professional care during the most critical moments of my life. I also extend heartfelt thanks to the dedicated staff at DACH Ayurvedic Hospital in Sri Lanka; your efforts during my recovery meant more than words can express.

To my friends, colleagues, and those who quietly stood by me with kind words and open hearts, thank you. Your support reminded me that I was not alone and that my journey mattered.

A special thank you goes to my readers. If this book finds its way into your hands, I hope my story offers strength, clarity, and inspiration. Whether you're facing a health challenge, navigating uncertainty, or seeking renewal, I want you to know that transformation is always possible.

This book is for every soul who chooses to hope over fear and who refuses to give up.

With deepest gratitude,

Channa A. G.

Table of Contents

Introduction: This Is Not Just My Story - It Could Be Yours Too 01

Chapter 1: The Moment Everything Changed 03

Chapter 2: Understanding the Message 15

Chapter 3: Accepting, Not Surrendering 27

Chapter 4: My Total Reset 37

Chapter 5: Learning to Let Go 53

Chapter 6: Building Better Habits 61

Chapter 7: Movement is Medicine 69

Chapter 8: Health is the First Wealth 75

Chapter 9: Purpose, Not Pressure 83

Chapter 10: My New Beginning 91

References 97

About the Author 99

Other Books by the Author 101

Stay Connected 103

Introduction: This Is Not Just My Story - It Could Be Yours Too

This book is about my journey through a life-altering experience, a stroke that challenged me not only physically but also mentally, emotionally, and spiritually. However, let me be clear: **this is not a story of someone who lost all physical ability and then miraculously regained it.** It's not just about muscles, medicine, or hospitals. It's about something deeper, how I transformed my entire life, inside and out.

When I suffered my stroke, I wasn't obese. I didn't have major health problems at the time. I was a husband, a father, and a postgraduate student pursuing a master's degree in the UK. On the surface, life was full of purpose. But underneath, I was neglecting my most important asset: my health.

This book is not fiction. Every word comes from lived experience. What I share here isn't meant to impress you; it's meant to inspire and support you. Because I believe that my experience can help others. You may not have had a stroke, but maybe you've faced burnout, chronic stress, poor health, or the quiet voice in your mind telling you to change before it's too late.

Throughout this book, I'll not only share what happened to me, but I'll also connect my experience with science-backed explanations. I believe that understanding the 'why' behind our struggles and recoveries brings confidence and clarity. You'll find references to medical research, neuroscience, lifestyle medicine, and mental health studies. Because when inspiration is supported by evidence, transformation becomes even more powerful.

Through these chapters, I will walk you through how I changed my life, mentally, physically, and emotionally. I'll talk about the wake-up call I received, the decisions I made, and how I began to build a life that was not just about surviving but thriving. I'll also share the struggles, the small victories, the shifts in mindset, and the habits that carried me forward.

Most importantly, I want to have a real conversation with you. About life. About health. About the purpose. About how fragile, yet powerful, we are. If you're willing to take this journey with me, I promise it won't just be about my healing, it could become the beginning of yours, too.

Because one truth echoes through every chapter of this book: **Health is the first wealth.** Without it, everything else fades. With it, anything is possible.

Welcome to *From Patient to Power: My Stroke Didn't Win.* Let this be the start of something new for you, too.

Chapter 1

The Moment Everything Changed

One Morning in June

It was a typical June morning in 2024. Like most weekdays, I was getting ready to drop my son off at school. The clock read around 6:15 a.m., and the cool air, about 15°C, brushed against the quiet of the early hours. Everything felt routine. I had already prepared my son's school uniform, and I went into the bathroom, as usual, to freshen up before heading out.

As I stood under the shower, something felt... off.

Suddenly, I noticed a strange heaviness on the left side of my body. My left arm and leg weren't moving the way I wanted them to. When I tried to lift my hand to wash my face, it came up, but very slowly, not like normal. It felt disconnected, as if my body and mind were no longer fully in sync. I remember thinking, *"Why isn't my hand working properly?"* It was the first moment I knew something was seriously wrong.

A wave of confusion and fear hit me.

But somehow, I stayed calm. I quietly unlocked the bathroom door, just in case, and continued washing myself slowly, doing what I could with the parts of my body that still worked. As soon as I finished, I stepped out and called for my wife.

My speech had already started to slur. My words weren't coming out clearly. I walked over to the mirror and smiled, hoping I was imagining things, but my smile gave it away. One side of my mouth had dropped. I was watching the signs unfold in real time.

And that's when it hit me:

I think I'm going to be paralysed.

I was terrified, but I didn't panic. I knew I had to act fast.

When the Doctor Becomes the Patient

As an Ayurvedic physician, I've treated many patients with paralysis. It's something I became very familiar with during my time in medical college, later while working in hospitals, and even through daily life at my own Ayurvedic practice. In fact, a large portion of the patients I've cared for over the years were paralysed. And thanks to Ayurveda, we've had great success in helping many of them regain their strength and independence.

So, for me, as a doctor, paralysis is not something new or unusual. I understand it clinically. I know the symptoms, the progression, and the treatment protocols by heart.

But this time, it was different.

This time... it was happening to me.

I remember thinking, *"If I become paralysed... what will happen?"* The fear wasn't just about the condition, it was about losing control. About what it would mean for my family, my future, and my purpose. I could already feel my left side weakening, and I wondered, *"Will I be completely paralysed in the next moment?"*

And then came another thought: *"How will I handle this, here, in a foreign country?"*

Back home in Sri Lanka, I would have had so many people around me, family, friends, and colleagues, ready to support me without hesitation. But here in the UK, at that moment, it felt like I had only one or two people I could truly rely on.

Still, one thing became very clear in my mind:
"This is not the time for me to be paralysed."
I have so much more to do in this life. I am not finished yet.

The Moment of Realisation

In that moment, I felt something that I believe everyone should experience, at least once, before they leave this world: The realisation that you are not finished.

Lying there, struggling to move, a wave of thoughts crashed over me. *"I'm not ready."*

I have a son, he's just eleven.
I have a wife, she depends on me for so many things.
They don't even know the passwords to our accounts or how to access our insurance plans. I hadn't handed over any of it. All those responsibilities, all those little details of life, I was still the one holding them all.

And now, I might not even get the chance to pass them on.

I've seen patients with minor symptoms suddenly deteriorate and pass away. I know how quickly things can change. One moment, you feel a little off: the next moment, it's over. As a doctor, I understood this medically. But now, as a patient, I felt it in my bones.

It's in moments like these that life teaches you what truly matters.
Not money.
Not titles.
But the people who count on you.
The work you haven't finished.
The words you haven't said.

That morning was no longer about dropping my son off at school. It became about understanding life, and how fragile, unfinished, and precious it truly is.

Recovery and Reflection

Around ten minutes later, most of my symptoms started to subside. My speech returned to normal, and my left hand and leg regained their usual strength. I felt much more stable, but there was still a lingering weakness on the left side of my body. My left hand couldn't grip anything as tightly as usual, and I started feeling a radiating pain from my left shoulder joint.

At that point, I called one of my very good friends who lived nearby. He came over immediately and advised me to call emergency services. He also took the responsibility of dropping my son off at school. My son was always excited to go to school, and he agreed to go with my friend, though I could still picture his face as he left.

He didn't say anything, but I could tell something was on his mind. A few days later, I asked him what he had been thinking. He told me that, at school, he often thought about what happened. My son knew that I had been treating patients with similar conditions for years, back in Sri Lanka. He had seen me work with paralysed patients in the hospital, but it was different for him when I became the patient. He wasn't ready to see me in that vulnerable position.

In the Hands of Others

My wife called emergency services, and within 30 minutes, the paramedics arrived. They were calm, professional, and kind, two women who had years of experience. They checked my blood pressure, tested my blood sugar, and then assessed the strength in my arms and hands.

One of the paramedics asked me to press against her hands and push with full strength, to see if both sides were working equally. That's when I realised my left side was still a bit weaker.

After the examination, they decided it was best to take me to the hospital. I could tell they knew exactly what they were doing. Their confidence and professionalism made me feel safe. Without their clinical knowledge, it would've been almost impossible, even for someone educated, to understand just how dangerous these "little" symptoms could be.

"I climbed into the ambulance, and my wife came along with me, sitting by my side during the ride. "On the way, I asked one of the paramedics, "Where are we going?"
She said gently, "We're taking you to Hull Royal Infirmary."

Then I heard her contact the hospital:
"We're bringing in a 39-year-old male with sudden left-sided weakness."

That moment stayed with me.

I have no identity beyond my age and symptoms. Just a 39-year-old man being taken to the hospital. It was a humbling moment. My ego vanished. I was simply someone in need of help. And I was ready to face whatever came next.

Facing the Truth

When we arrived at the hospital, the stroke consultant and his team were already waiting for me. That gave me a deep sense of confidence. It felt different from what I'd experienced in my home country, more coordinated, more immediate.

The consultant introduced himself with calm authority, and his assistant also introduced herself warmly. They moved quickly but respectfully, never making me feel like just another case.

I was immediately taken for a CT scan. After reviewing the images, the doctor returned and said, "The CT looks normal, but based on your symptoms, we need to do an MRI to be sure."

Not long after, the MRI was done. A little while later, I was told the result:

"The MRI confirms you've had a left cerebellar infarct."

I had suffered a stroke.

Even though I had already suspected something was wrong, hearing those words hit me differently. This was now confirmed. Real. Named. Documented.

The Next Steps

After confirming the stroke, the doctors explained that they needed to do further investigations to understand why this had happened. They took more blood samples for additional tests and assured me that they would follow up once the results were ready.

The consultant then looked me in the eye and said something I'll never forget:
"You are at very high risk of having another stroke within the next couple of days, and if it happens, it could be much more severe than this one."

That moment felt like a personal alarm bell, loud and clear. A warning I couldn't ignore.

He advised me not to drive for at least 30 days. He also prescribed medication to manage my condition and reduce the risk of another event.

Once everything was explained and I was medically stable, they discharged me with clear instructions: If anything changes, call emergency services immediately.

Everything, from scans to diagnosis to discharge, happened within half a day. Just like that, it was over. No hospital admission. No overnight stay.

I left the hospital quietly, alone in thought. My wife and I took a taxi home.

Take the Message the First Time

This is one of the most important lessons I've learned: many people get a warning before a major stroke, often in the form of a mini-stroke, or what doctors call a TIA. But too often, these signs are misunderstood or ignored. That moment of weakness, slurred speech, or dizziness? People brush it off. "Maybe I didn't sleep enough," or "I'm just stressed," they say. But this thinking can be dangerously wrong.

In my case, it wasn't just a TIA. What was first called a mini stroke turned out to be an actual stroke, confirmed by the MRI. While others may get a warning, I had already crossed the line.

The message my body was sending wasn't just a whisper, it was a full alarm.

And like any alarm in life, it only helps if you respond the first time.

Understanding the Warning: The Significance of a Mini-Stroke

Experiencing a TIA is not just a fleeting health scare; it's a critical warning sign. According to the Mayo Clinic, about one in three individuals who experience a TIA will subsequently have a stroke, with approximately half of these strokes occurring within a year. The risk is particularly high within the first 48 hours following a TIA. (Mayo Clinic, 2024)

This underscores the importance of immediate medical evaluation and intervention after a TIA. Prompt treatment can significantly reduce the risk of a subsequent, potentially more severe stroke. Healthcare professionals often use the ABCD score to assess the short-term risk of stroke after a TIA, considering factors such as age, blood pressure, clinical features, duration of symptoms, and diabetes. (American Stroke Association, 2025)

Recognising and responding to the signs of a TIA can be lifesaving. It's a pivotal moment that calls for reflection, lifestyle adjustments, and adherence to medical advice to mitigate future risks.

Chapter 2

Understanding the Message

Early Eating Habits and Daily Routine

When I experienced my stroke, I had been living in the UK for just about a year. That moment forced me to reflect deeply on the life I had led up until then, especially my lifestyle habits.

In my younger years, especially up to age 20 or 22, I was quite slim and maintained a body weight appropriate for my height. I didn't think too much about health back then. I was just like most young people, active, busy, and burning energy quickly. I ate the way most Sri Lankans do: three main meals a day, built around rice, vegetables, and either meat or fish. In the mornings, I usually had bread, hoppers, or roti. Lunch was always rice and curry, and dinner followed a similar pattern, sometimes hoppers, sometimes fried rice, depending on what was available.

Mealtimes were also regular, breakfast around 7 a.m., lunch at 1 p.m., and dinner around 8 p.m. This rhythm was common among many Sri Lankans, and it felt normal.

But there's something we aren't often taught growing up: as we get older, our bodies change, and so should our habits. In our education, we weren't taught that eating the same way through life could eventually catch up with us. I used to think, "I'll change my eating habits when I'm in my 50s or 60s, when

I start feeling the effects." But I didn't realise that change needs to start much earlier, even in our younger years.

After the age of 20, certainly by 25, things began to change. Our metabolism slows down with age, and if we keep eating the same quantity and type of food without adjusting our habits, the body starts to store excess fat. That's exactly what happened to me. I began to gain weight in my late 20s, and by the time I reached 30, I had a noticeable increase in fat accumulation.

It's not just in Sri Lanka; people in many other countries also focus heavily on flour-based foods, especially bakery items like bread and buns, as well as junk food such as burgers and pizza. These eating habits are like rice-heavy diets in that they can all contribute to weight gain when not balanced properly.

According to recent global research, approximately 43% of adults worldwide are classified as overweight, and 16% live with obesity, a condition that continues to rise largely due to poor dietary habits and sedentary lifestyles (WHO, 2023). These figures reflect a global trend where the shift toward processed foods, sugary beverages, and reduced physical activity is significantly contributing to the obesity epidemic. The World Obesity Federation (2024) also projects that by

2035, over 1.5 billion adults will be living with obesity, with a notable increase in low- and middle-income countries.

However, the key to addressing obesity is not just about what we eat, but also how we approach food. Regardless of nationality, cultural food traditions can still accommodate healthier food choices. With improved awareness and mindful eating practices, anyone can adapt their meals to be more nutritious. This highlights the importance of not only focusing on the quality of food but also on portion control, meal timing, and balance, which are essential in managing weight and improving health.

After entering university, I gained knowledge about diet control, healthy food choices, and how food affects health according to Ayurveda. I learned about suitable foods for different stages of life and the importance of adjusting our diets as we age. My wife and I discussed how we could apply these dietary principles to our own lives.

During our university years, we had the time to focus on our diet and maintain control over what we ate. However, as life progressed, with business responsibilities, raising children, and managing day-to-day tasks, I found it increasingly difficult to stick to my diet plan. Despite my best efforts, I wasn't always able to maintain the discipline I had during those university years.

Though I managed to maintain a weight of around 70-72 kg, at a height of 164 cm, my BMI indicated that I was overweight.

Before coming to the UK, my life in Sri Lanka was extremely busy. Between running my business and fulfilling various responsibilities, I often didn't get enough rest. Most nights, I had frequent gatherings, sometimes with friends, sometimes with business partners, and often with my charity group. These gatherings usually took place at my home and often continued late into the night, sometimes until 11 or 12, and on occasion, even into the early hours of the next day.

Although I was not a smoker and didn't consume hard liquor, I did occasionally have beer or wine in limited amounts. However, during these social events, my friends and partners would often drink, and as part of the social habit, I would eat more snacks, which we call "bites" in Sri Lanka. These typically included deep-fried pork or chicken, fried rice, fried vegetables, and chips, all rich in oil and unhealthy ingredients.

This became a regular pattern for me, and over time, I developed a habit of consuming these types of foods more frequently than I should have. Coupled with the late nights, I often slept less than six hours, which affected my overall health and energy levels.

In my personal experience, inadequate sleep and frequent consumption of unhealthy foods, particularly late at night, led to noticeable changes in my cholesterol levels. Research supports this observation, indicating that sleep deprivation can elevate total cholesterol and low-density lipoprotein (LDL) cholesterol levels while reducing high-density lipoprotein (HDL) cholesterol levels (Chaput et al., 2014). Additionally, consuming high-fat foods or eating at irregular times, such as late at night, has been linked to worsened lipid profiles, leading to higher cholesterol levels (Horne & Pankhurst, 2017). Consequently, I had to initiate medication to manage my cholesterol effectively.

Moving to the UK and Adapting to a New Lifestyle

In mid-2023, I moved to the UK to pursue my further studies in business management. I chose to do a master's in business because I wanted to gain deeper knowledge in the field and strengthen my ability to manage and grow my ventures. After relocating, my daily routine began to shift. I became more conscious about my diet and lifestyle habits. I started jogging regularly and made a real effort to control my eating patterns.

Living in the UK, especially while commuting to London for my studies, brought more physical activity into my life. I often used the train to travel, and I walked more, especially between stations and the university. Unlike in Sri Lanka, where my schedule was constantly packed with work and social commitments, here I found more free time. This change allowed me to be more active and focused on my well-being. As a result, I lost around 2 to 3 kilograms and maintained my weight at around 68 kg.

Balancing Diet Between Two Worlds

While living in the UK, I significantly reduced my rice intake and tried to follow a lower-carb diet as much as possible. Although I occasionally ate rice and high-carb foods out of habit, I kept it under much better control than I did in Sri Lanka. However, during this period, I travelled to Sri Lanka three times for short vacations.

Each time I returned home, my routine shifted dramatically. I attended frequent gatherings, and I slipped back into my old food habits, high in carbs, oily dishes, and irregular mealtimes. About two months before my stroke, I was in Sri Lanka again. My daily routine became hectic during those two weeks, filled with business work and social functions. As a result, my total cholesterol and triglyceride levels spiked significantly during that time. The combination of unhealthy eating and a busy, unbalanced schedule set the stage for a serious health warning that was soon to come.

Reflection on My Health Habits: A Wake-Up Call

After coming to the UK, I spent two months adjusting to my new life. During this time, I gained more insight into how my daily habits and routines directly impacted my health. Although I wasn't obese and didn't have any severe medical issues at that point, my cholesterol levels began to rise over time. I managed to control it with some medication, but the reality was clear: my lifestyle was contributing to these problems.

This experience made me reflect on the dangers of consistently making poor health choices. If someone continues to eat unhealthy foods, consume excessive sugar, and neglect exercise, the long-term impact can be devastating. The cumulative effect of these habits can lead to serious health issues like high cholesterol, heart disease, and even stroke.

Two months after adjusting to life in the UK, I experienced a stroke, a direct consequence of all these past habits. It was a wake-up call that made me realise just how damaging these lifestyle choices could be. Every choice, big or small, shapes our health over time, and in my case, it had reached a point where the consequences were no longer avoidable.

Realisation That Success Means Nothing Without Health

After experiencing my stroke, I had a powerful realisation, everything I had achieved, all my success, meant nothing without my health. That moment made it clear: I needed to completely transform my life. I had the knowledge and experience already, especially through my background in Ayurveda, yet I wasn't truly applying it to myself.

It was time to return to a more natural and healthier lifestyle. I knew I had to change my diet, my habits, and my entire daily routine. At age 40, I still have so much to live for. My son is still young, and I want to be there for him, for his future, for his milestones.

I also asked myself: If I have everything, money, property, wealth, but not my health, what does it all mean? Without health, nothing truly matters. But if you are healthy, you can do anything, you can achieve your goals, chase your dreams, and live a full, purposeful life. Health must come first. Everything else follows.

This was the moment I truly understood: I must take control now, before another stroke happens. There's no more room for delay; my life depends on the changes I make today.

Chapter 3

Accepting, Not Surrendering

The stroke didn't just shake my body; it cracked open my entire way of seeing the world. One moment, life felt familiar. Next, I was plunged into uncertainty, silence, and stillness. But in that stillness, something essential was revealed: a raw, undeniable truth.

Everything had to change.

This wasn't about being a victim or a warrior. It wasn't about winning or losing. It was about becoming. I already knew. I already had the tools. But now, I had something even more powerful: the reason.

This was not the end of my story. It was the messy, humbling, courageous beginning of a new chapter, one rooted in acceptance, but never in surrender.

Accepting the Diagnosis, Not the Defeat

When the doctor sat down and said the words, *"You've had a stroke",* time slowed. My breath caught. Even with my background in Ayurveda and years of health education and professional experience, nothing could have fully prepared me for that moment.

I felt a swirl of emotions: disbelief, fear, shame, sadness. I kept thinking, *how could this happen to me? I should have known better.* But health isn't always about learning.

Sometimes it's about noticing, and I hadn't noticed the small signs. I'd been too busy, too focused on the external world, and not present enough with my inner signals.

Still, as the initial shock began to settle, something deeper emerged: acceptance.

I didn't argue with the diagnosis. I didn't slip into denial or anger. I allowed myself to sit with the truth. And that became my first step toward healing.

Let me be clear, acceptance is not giving up. It's the opposite. It is an act of bravery. It's facing your truth, however uncomfortable, and saying, *"Yes. This is real. But it is not the end of me."*

I accepted the reality of what had happened, but I refused to accept defeat. A diagnosis is just a snapshot in time. It may describe a moment, but it does not dictate the entire story. I chose to use it as a turning point, not a finish line.

Rebuilding My Mindset and Outlook

In the days that followed, I found myself in deep reflection. The physical fatigue was real, but so was the mental clarity. I began asking powerful questions:

- Who do I want to become from here?
- What kind of life do I truly want to lead?

- What will I no longer tolerate, from myself or my circumstances?

I realised that mindset is the soil in which healing takes root. Without it, even the best treatments may not bloom. A strong mind builds a strong body, and that strength doesn't come from pretending you're okay. It comes from choosing to grow, even when everything feels uncertain.

I chose not to rebuild out of fear, guilt, or pressure. I rebuilt from calm clarity. I returned to the practices I had once taught others but hadn't always fully embodied myself. I began journaling every day, not just about what I did, but how I felt. I meditated not for performance, but for presence. I reconnected with the Ayurvedic wisdom that had once lit my path.

Every day became a reset. Every meal, every breath, every bedtime ritual is intentional. Purposeful. Not perfect, but aligned.

I wasn't trying to be who I was before. I was trying to become someone new, someone wiser, more balanced, more present.

The Beginning of Inner Strength

There is a quiet strength that comes when you stop fighting your reality and start working with it. That strength doesn't roar. It doesn't shout. It whispers, *"You are still here. You are still capable. Start from here."*

This strength wasn't about lifting heavy weights or powering through exhaustion. It was about showing up for myself. Consistently. Gently. With grace.

Even on the days when fatigue came like a wave or fear crept in like a shadow, I anchored myself in a deeper purpose, my son, my family, my mission in life. These weren't just ideas anymore. They were the reason I kept getting up. The reason I kept going.

Ayurveda teaches us about the balance between the body, mind, and spirit. I began to consciously cultivate sattva, the state of harmony and clarity. I simplified everything: my routines, my thoughts, my environment. I removed what drained me and leaned into what nourished me.

This wasn't about control. It was about choosing peace over chaos, intention over impulse.

Choosing Not to Be a Victim

The most powerful decision I made was this: I would not be a victim of my circumstances.

It would have been easy to fall into that story: *"Why me?"* Easy to point fingers at stress, overwork, pressure, genetics, and fate. But that path only leads to more suffering, and I needed every ounce of energy for healing, not blame.

So instead, I chose to say: *"Yes, this happened. But I'm still here. And I still have a choice."*

That choice was everything.

I leaned into gratitude. I looked at what I still had: my mind, my spirit, my willpower. I thought of others who never got the chance to wake up and try again. I had been gifted a second chance, and I wasn't going to waste it.

Not surrendering didn't mean pretending everything was fine. It meant refusing to let my pain define me. It meant using the pain as fuel, not a cage.

From Acceptance to Action

Acceptance is not passive. It is the doorway to transformation. But stepping through that doorway? That requires action.

I got serious about my diet, choosing foods that weren't just tasty, but truly healing. I simplified my meals, focused on digestibility, and listened to how my body responded. I restructured my sleep and committed to deep rest, knowing recovery thrives on stillness as much as movement.

I reconnected with my body in new ways, not through punishing workouts, but through joyful, conscious movement. Nature walks, breathwork, and yoga with deep presence. I began treating my body not as a machine to be pushed, but as a sacred vessel to be cared for.

Most importantly, I started living what I knew. All the Ayurvedic knowledge, the mindset strategies, and the life experience, I brought them to life. In real time. With real discipline.

That's when the shift happened. I started feeling like myself again, not the old version, but a wiser, calmer, more grounded version. A version I could be proud of.

A New Identity, Rooted in Strength

Today, I don't introduce myself as a stroke survivor. I introduce myself as someone who chose to rise.

This chapter of my life is not about illness. It's about ownership. About taking responsibility for my choices, my healing, and my path forward.

I have accepted my past. I've made peace with what happened. But I will never surrender my future to fear, to complacency, or to regret.

My new identity is not just built on what I overcame. It's built on how I responded. And that's the message I want to leave with you:

We don't get to choose every storm. But we do get to choose who we become in the aftermath.

Let your challenges become your compass. Let acceptance become your power. And never, ever surrender to anything less than the life you deserve.

Chapter 4

My Total Reset

A Brief Journey to Sri Lanka for Natural Healing

After discussing my condition with consultants at Hull Hospital, I decided to travel to Sri Lanka to begin my preferred course of treatment through Ayurveda. Despite the initial hospital care, I continued to experience discomfort, pain on my left side, a sense of unsteadiness, occasional weakness, and a persistent lack of balance. In the UK, further investigations and treatment options would take more time, and I didn't want to wait. I felt I needed a more holistic approach, something that addressed not just my symptoms but my entire well-being.

To make this possible, I obtained permission from my university to temporarily step away from my studies. They were understanding and supportive, which gave me peace of mind as I planned my healing journey.

So, in June, on my 40th birthday, I flew back to Sri Lanka, not just to heal, but to reset. It was a symbolic moment: entering a new decade of life and choosing to reclaim it through the healing principles I deeply believe in.

Sharing My Condition: A Wake-Up Call for Others

When I arrived in Sri Lanka, most of my friends, colleagues, and extended family were shocked. I hadn't informed many people before leaving the UK, except for a few close relatives who knew the real reason for my sudden visit. So, when they saw me in person, still recovering, visibly affected, and moving carefully, they were stunned. For many, it was the first time they realised something serious had happened to me.

The news spread quickly, and their reactions were full of concern, confusion, and disbelief. They couldn't believe that I, someone they viewed as energetic, successful, and always on the move, had suffered a stroke. Many of them told me they thought I was in perfect health. But that's the danger, external appearances don't always reflect what's happening inside.

What surprised me even more was how my experience became a wake-up call for them. Many of my friends and colleagues admitted that their lifestyles were even worse than mine: more stress, less sleep, poor diets, and no exercise. Seeing what had happened to me made them stop and reflect. They began asking questions about their health, some even deciding to get medical checkups and consider healthier routines.

It was a deeply emotional experience for all of us. My situation served as a shock not just to me, but to my entire circle. I hadn't expected to become an example like this, but if my story could help others act before it's too late, then it had a greater purpose.

Light Panchakarma Therapies, Herbal Decoctions, and Lifestyle Balancing

During my time in Sri Lanka, I decided to begin my recovery with Ayurvedic treatment, a path I deeply believed in, both professionally and personally. I own an Ayurvedic hospital in Sri Lanka, and after discussing my condition in detail with the medical team there, including senior physicians and my wife, who also has deep knowledge in the field, we carefully planned a holistic treatment approach tailored specifically to my needs.

It was an emotional and humbling experience. Being treated in my hospital by staff who knew me not just as a practitioner or employer, but as a patient, created a strange, vulnerable feeling. Many of my team members felt a bit uncomfortable at first; they weren't used to seeing me in this role. But over time, that discomfort turned into care, dedication, and genuine support. They treated me with deep respect and compassion, which made a huge difference in my healing process.

Together, we designed a treatment series based on classical Ayurvedic texts. We prepared personalised herbal decoctions using traditional formulations, aimed at balancing my aggravated doshas, particularly targeting vata imbalance, which often plays a major role in neurological and post-stroke conditions. These internal medicines were supported by external Panchakarma-inspired therapies that focused on calming the nervous system, improving circulation, and reducing pain (Manohar et al., 2021; Patwardhan et al., 2005).

One of the key treatments was Shirodhara, a deeply soothing procedure where warm, medicated oil is gently poured in a continuous stream over the forehead. This therapy had a profound calming effect on my mind and body, helping reduce anxiety, improve sleep, and support mental clarity. I also underwent gentle oil applications (Abhyanga), followed by herbal steam therapy, and a light cleansing protocol suited to my post-stroke recovery state.

Over about one and a half months, I began to feel significant improvements. The constant pain and heaviness on the left side of my body started to fade. The unsteadiness and weakness I had been struggling with slowly decreased. More importantly, I began to feel like myself again, clearer, more focused, and stronger both physically and mentally.

By the end of my Ayurvedic treatment phase, I felt renewed and confident in my recovery journey. This experience was more than just a physical healing, it was a return to my roots, a reconnection to the wisdom of Ayurveda, and a reminder that even as a healer, I, too, must be willing to receive care, follow discipline, and allow time for full restoration.

The Beginning of My Full Lifestyle Overhaul

After completing my Ayurvedic treatment in Sri Lanka and starting to feel stronger both physically and emotionally, I returned to the UK two months later. I had to complete my master's degree and submit my dissertation on time. Thankfully, I was granted a two-week extension by the university, which gave me just enough breathing room to settle back in and focus on my academic responsibilities.

But more importantly, I came back with a renewed mindset. I knew that I couldn't return to the same lifestyle that had led me to a stroke. This was the beginning of a complete reset. I realised that my earlier failures, ignoring rest, eating carelessly, neglecting consistent physical activity, were not just small mistakes; they were choices that had nearly cost me everything. It was time to take full ownership of my life.

From that point forward, I committed myself to building a new kind of balance. This time, it wasn't just about achieving success in studies or business. It was about creating a sustainable, healthy life where my mind, body, and spirit could grow together.

My past experiences, combined with my Ayurvedic medical background and new business education, gave me a powerful foundation to create meaningful change. In this book, I want to share exactly how I redesigned my daily routines, how I applied both ancient wisdom and modern tools, and how I turned a health crisis into a turning point. I'm not just writing about what happened, I'm showing what I did, what I'm doing now, and what anyone can do to transform their own life, step by step.

I Stopped Sugar and White Flour Completely

Food has always played a central role in my life, and, as I've come to realise, also in many of my health challenges. Over the years, I learned that what we eat must change as we age. Our dietary needs at 20 are not the same at 40, and they certainly won't be at 60. Especially after the age of 35 or 40, we must become more intentional and disciplined about our food choices.

One of the most transformative decisions I made was to eliminate sugar and white flour from my diet entirely. Many people think avoiding sugar means just skipping desserts or sweets. But the reality is far more complex. Sugar is hidden in countless everyday foods, especially those made with refined wheat flour like bread, roti, pasta, buns, and chapati. These foods may not taste sweet, but they trigger rapid spikes in blood sugar and insulin levels, which over time contribute to inflammation, fatigue, weight gain, and metabolic syndrome. Leading researchers have described added sugar as a "toxic" substance in the modern diet, linked to a wide range of non-communicable diseases, including obesity, diabetes, and cardiovascular disease (Lustig, Schmidt, & Brindis, 2012).

To truly understand how my body responded to food, I began using a continuous glucose monitor (CGM). This was a game-changer. I learned that even seemingly healthy or neutral foods could cause sharp blood sugar spikes. A 2015 study published in *Cell* confirmed that individuals respond very differently to the same foods; what's healthy for one person might be harmful to another (Zeevi et al., 2015). This real-time data helped me personalise my eating habits, making choices that supported healing and eliminated silent harm.

One key lesson I've learned, and I want others to understand, is that most of us eat far more than we need. Many people think they can "burn it off" by going to the gym or walking more, but they underestimate how hard it is to burn off excess calories, especially from sugar and refined carbs. It's far more effective to manage what goes into your body in the first place.

Your diet is either your best medicine or your slowest poison. For me, cutting out sugar and white flour wasn't a diet trend; it was a survival decision. And it changed everything.

Started Regular Exercise and Joined a Gym

About six months after my stroke, I consulted with my stroke specialist in the UK to discuss whether it was safe for me to start exercising again. With his approval and some guidance on how to ease into physical activity safely, I decided to begin a structured workout routine. This marked another key turning point in my recovery.

I joined a local gym and began to train consistently, but I approached it very differently than most people do. Many believe they can simply "burn off" unhealthy meals at the gym. However, I quickly realised that exercise alone is not enough. Unless you also manage your food intake, you're only addressing half the problem. In fact, without controlling your diet, even hours in the gym won't deliver the results you're hoping for.

Because I was already following a low-carb, clean diet, I didn't need to do intense cardio or high-volume workouts to maintain or improve my health. My goal was to regain strength, improve balance, and enhance overall energy, not to punish my body.

Thankfully, I had a close friend who had been training in the same gym for over five years and was very disciplined with both his workouts and his diet. He offered to guide me. Based on his advice, I focused on muscle-building exercises rather than just cardio. He recommended a simple but effective plan: train for one hour, three times a week, concentrating mainly on the upper body, chest, shoulders, and back, as well as supporting lower-body exercises. He also encouraged me to use the treadmill for 20 to 30 minutes to build endurance and warm up my muscles.

In addition to gym workouts, whenever I had extra time and the weather allowed, I went jogging outdoors, usually around 4 to 5 kilometres. This combination of light strength training and cardiovascular movement helped me improve my physical balance and confidence without exhausting myself.

This routine didn't leave me feeling drained or overwhelmed. It energised me. I started to notice improvements in my mood, strength, and focus. The muscle tone in my body began to return, and I felt more in control of myself physically and mentally.

Now, I can confidently say I am in better shape than I was before my stroke. Exercise has become more than just a recovery tool; it is now a key part of my lifestyle. It keeps me grounded, helps me stay positive, and reminds me every day that I am stronger than my past.

Prioritising Quality Sleep and Deep Rest

Sleep is one of the most essential yet often overlooked aspects of our health. Before my stroke, I didn't fully grasp how much sleep truly impacted my body. I had always been a busy person, juggling multiple responsibilities between my business, family, and social commitments. As a result, I regularly sacrificed sleep to keep up with everything. But I learned the hard way that a lack of sleep can have profound consequences on both physical and mental health.

When I was not getting enough rest, I noticed that my blood triglyceride levels would rise significantly. This is a major risk factor for stroke, and seeing this correlation between my poor sleep habits and rising health markers was a wake-up call. I realised that I needed to take sleep as seriously as I took my diet and exercise. Research confirms that insufficient sleep is associated with increased risks of cardiovascular disease, metabolic disorders, and impaired immune function (Walker, 2017).

Now, I make it a point to get 7 to 8 hours of quality sleep every night. It's not just about the quantity of sleep, but also the quality. To monitor this, I use an AI-powered ring that tracks my sleep patterns and provides data on how well I'm resting. This technology has been incredibly helpful in understanding how my body reacts to different sleep conditions, like temperature, sleep stages, and how much deep sleep I'm getting. It's given me insight into areas where I can improve my sleep hygiene and achieve better rest.

One key realisation I had during this process is how many people, including myself, often waste time on distractions, television, computers, and especially mobile phones. These activities can significantly reduce the amount of sleep we get. The blue light emitted by screens disrupts the production of melatonin, the hormone responsible for regulating sleep, and this can make it harder to fall asleep and stay asleep.

If we can control these habits and make a conscious effort to limit screen time before bed, we can reclaim our sleep. Establishing a nighttime routine that includes winding down, whether it's reading a book, meditating, or simply reflecting on the day, can go a long way in improving the quality of our rest.

Having quality sleep is one of the most powerful tools for maintaining good health. It's essential not only for physical recovery but also for mental clarity, emotional balance, and overall well-being. I now prioritise sleep just as much as I prioritise my food and exercise. I understand that without proper sleep, all the other health practices I follow won't be as effective. So, sleep has become a fundamental pillar of my new lifestyle.

The Path to Transformation

As I look back on the past few months, it's clear that the changes I made weren't just about a physical transformation; they were about reshaping my entire approach to life. The combination of Ayurvedic healing, dietary changes, regular exercise, and prioritising sleep has had a profound impact on my health. I feel stronger, more balanced, and more in tune with my body than ever before.

But this journey is far from over. It's an ongoing process of refining, learning, and growing. The lessons I've learned about the importance of balance, the power of consistency, and the need for self-compassion will continue to guide me in the years to come.

I've come to realise that health isn't just the absence of illness; it's a dynamic state of well-being that requires attention and intention. By making small, consistent changes every day, we can all take control of our health and create a life that feels both fulfilling and vibrant. My transformation has only just begun, and I am committed to staying on this path of renewal, understanding that true strength comes from within.

This chapter of my journey has been a reset, a new beginning, not just for my body, but for my mind, heart, and spirit. And as I continue forward, I know that I'm building a foundation for a healthier, more purposeful life.

Chapter 5

Learning to Let Go

In the aftermath of my stroke, a powerful realisation began to take shape: true healing wasn't just about repairing my body. The most transformative part of my recovery was learning how to let go: letting go of the past, of regrets, of the relentless expectations I had placed on myself, and of the constant pressure to always be in control. These emotional burdens had quietly shaped my lifestyle for years, and they had taken a toll I could no longer ignore.

Letting Go of Regrets, Perfectionism, and Pressure

For much of my life, I lived with a silent script in my mind, one that demanded progress, perfection, and productivity. I was always reaching for the next goal, pushing through fatigue, convincing myself that slowing down meant falling behind. This constant drive to "do more" came with a price: an overwhelming inner pressure and a deep fear of failure.

Before the stroke, I wasn't the kind of person to dwell on emotions or miss people easily. But I was someone who overthought things and worried a lot. I didn't always express it, but it showed up in other ways. Unanswered messages. Decisions are made too quickly. Constant thoughts of what I could've done better. These weren't big regrets, more like mental clutter that never switched off. Looking back, I can see how that quiet, ongoing pressure slowly wore me down and may have played a role in what happened to my body.

It was only after everything stopped, after life forced me to pause, that I began to truly reflect. Letting go wasn't about giving up. It was about releasing the mental and emotional clutter that no longer served me. I had to confront the perfectionism that had subtly dominated my thinking. For too long, I believed that mistakes defined me. That any slip was a failure. But in truth, perfectionism was a cage, one I had built myself.

The moment I stopped judging myself for every mistake, something shifted. I felt a kind of freedom I hadn't experienced in years. Letting go of the need to always get it right made space for something deeper, true healing.

Learning to Forgive Yourself and Others

One of the most important lessons I've learned is how much we simply don't see until we do. Back then, I didn't realise how much I was pushing past my limits: delaying rest, ignoring small warning signs, and putting everything else ahead of my well-being. It wasn't out of carelessness; it was just the pace I was used to. I wasn't blaming myself, but I could finally see how those choices added up over time. Recognising that was a quiet turning point. It brought clarity, and with it, the beginning of real change.

But forgiveness is not about forgetting or excusing. It's about releasing. I had to accept that I was doing the best I could with the awareness I had at the time. That simple truth allowed me to start again with compassion instead of criticism. Forgiving myself was not a one-time act, it was a slow unfolding, a practice I had to return to daily.

Equally important was my relationship with forgiveness. I've never been someone who holds onto hurt for long. I don't keep things buried in my heart or replay old arguments in my head. But after the stroke, something shifted, and I found myself letting go even faster. Sometimes, I didn't even stop to process it fully; I just didn't see the point in carrying anything heavy. It wasn't about ignoring the pain or pretending it didn't matter, it was about valuing peace over pride. Forgiveness became simple, quiet, and instinctive, a way of moving forward without carrying unnecessary weight.

Emotional Healing and Its Impact on Recovery

As I gradually released these emotional burdens, something surprising happened: I began to heal faster. My physical symptoms started improving more rapidly, my mind became clearer, and my energy returned in ways I hadn't expected. It was a clear sign that healing isn't just physical, it's emotional, psychological, and deeply personal.

Our emotions aren't just invisible thoughts; they are experiences that live in the body. Chronic stress, unresolved anger, and lingering guilt can manifest physically, raising blood pressure, disrupting sleep, weakening immunity, and more. I began to understand that emotional health isn't a "bonus" in recovery; it's a cornerstone.

Letting go of perfection, pressure, and pain helped bring balance back into my life. I stopped needing to be in control of everything. I started accepting that life unfolds with both uncertainty and beauty, and that peace is found not in controlling the chaos, but in learning to move with it.

The Real Strength in Surrender

I used to think that strength was about endurance, pushing through, standing tall, showing no weakness. But I've come to learn that real strength is found in surrender. It takes courage to admit you're tired. It takes resilience to start again with gentleness instead of grit. And it takes deep self-awareness to say: "This no longer serves me, and I'm ready to let it go."

Letting go has allowed me to create space for rest, for joy, for new perspectives. It has deepened my connection with those I love and helped me reconnect with the version of myself I had long forgotten: a person who values presence over perfection, peace over performance.

This isn't a lesson you learn once. Letting go is a daily practice. Sometimes, it's letting go of a harsh thought. Other times, it's letting go of control. Each day offers a small opportunity to unburden yourself and return to what matters.

And so, I've learned that the most powerful step in healing isn't always treatment or therapy, it's the moment we decide to release what no longer belongs. That's when transformation begins. That's when we truly begin to live again.

Chapter 6

Building Better Habits

The biggest truth I've learned on this journey is that healing isn't just about one big moment; it's about the small, daily steps that add up over time. Big breakthroughs are built on consistent action, not sudden inspiration. And that's exactly what this chapter is about: how I built better habits, day by day, that reshaped my life, my health, and my mindset.

Establishing a Powerful Daily Routine

After returning from Sri Lanka and settling back into the UK, I knew that the structure I had created during my recovery couldn't be left behind. If I wanted lasting change, I had to carry those habits into my everyday life. That meant building a strong daily routine that supported both my physical health and mental clarity.

Mornings became sacred. I started each day early, often before sunrise, with a short meditation to ground myself. Just five to ten minutes of silence helped me connect with my breath and set my intentions for the day. This was followed by light stretching or a brisk walk, just enough to wake up my body gently.

Then came a powerful ritual: my homemade energy-boosting drink. I combined Amla (Indian gooseberry) and Turmeric, both known for their anti-inflammatory and antioxidant properties, into a warm tonic. This simple blend helped me feel refreshed, alert, and energised, without relying on caffeine. It became a cornerstone of my mornings, and over time, I truly felt the difference in my stamina and focus.

I also became very intentional about how I managed my time. Instead of reacting to the day, I planned it. I blocked out time for meals, for exercise, for work, and most importantly, for rest. My phone wasn't the first thing I checked in the morning anymore. Instead, I gave myself time to be present before getting swept into the digital world. That single shift alone gave me a sense of control I never had before.

Building a routine wasn't just about being organised, it was about reclaiming my power. Every day that I followed through on my commitments, I felt more grounded, more focused, and more alive.

Sticking to Your New Eating Habits

Changing my diet was one of the most critical parts of my transformation. But more important than changing it was sticking to it. In the past, I'd made dietary changes before, but they never lasted. This time was different. I wasn't doing it to hit a goal weight or look a certain way, I was doing it to save my life and keep my mind sharp. That shift in motivation made all the difference.

I committed to eating only two meals a day. Not because of any trendy diet, but because I'd observed how my body functioned best with simplicity and discipline. My meals were based on clean protein, like fish or eggs, healthy fats like avocado or olive oil, and plenty of vegetables. I avoided all processed food, and especially sugar and refined carbohydrates.

Instead of thinking about what I was "missing out" on, I focused on how I felt: lighter, clearer, more focused. I wasn't bloated anymore. My energy levels were stable. I didn't crash in the afternoon like I used to. Food became fuel, not an emotional crutch.

And when cravings came, because they always do, I had strategies. I drank warm water with lemon, went for a short walk, or simply reminded myself of why I started. The goal wasn't to be perfect, but to stay consistent.

Removing Sugar and Flour Permanently

One of the biggest turning points in my recovery was realising how harmful sugar and white flour were, not just for my body, but for my brain. They caused inflammation, energy crashes, mood swings, and even affected my sleep. Research supports this connection: diets high in refined sugar and white flour have been shown to increase inflammation and negatively impact both brain function and mood regulation (Kris-Etherton et al., 2021). Through careful tracking (including using a continuous glucose monitor), I saw firsthand how even a small bite of bread, or a sugary snack would spike my blood sugar and leave me feeling unwell.

So, I made the decision: no more sugar, no more flour. This wasn't temporary. It wasn't a "diet." It was a new standard for how I wanted to live. And with that decision, everything became easier. I didn't have to debate with myself every time I saw a croissant or a slice of cake. The rule was clear, and that clarity gave me freedom.

I started preparing most of my meals at home and explored new recipes that aligned with my values. I carried healthy snacks when I travelled. And when I was invited to gatherings or parties, I simply made mindful choices, selecting healthier options from what was available. At first, people were surprised, but over time, they respected my discipline. Some even felt inspired to make changes in their own lives.

This wasn't about being strict for the sake of it. It was about honouring my body and protecting my brain from another stroke. Every time I said no to sugar and flour, I was saying yes to my future.

How Consistency, Not Motivation, Changed My Body and Brain

Here's a truth many people don't talk about: you won't always feel motivated. Motivation fades. It comes and goes with your mood, your energy, and your circumstances. But what doesn't fade is consistency. That's what creates real change.

I didn't go to the gym three or four times a week because I was always motivated. I went because I committed myself. I didn't stick to my eating habits because I felt strong every day. I did it because I created a rhythm that made staying on track feel more natural than falling off. I didn't meditate each morning because I always woke up calm. I did it because I knew how easily my mind could slip without that anchor.

Over time, those small daily actions rewired my brain. Neuroscience calls it neuroplasticity, the brain's ability to change based on repeated behaviour. And I experienced it firsthand. I became calmer, more focused, and emotionally stronger. I no longer needed willpower to resist temptation; it simply didn't appeal to me anymore.

This consistency helped me build not just a healthier body, but a more resilient mind. And with every passing day, those habits became who I was, not something I had to force, but something I naturally lived.

Small Steps, Stronger Self

Building better habits was the foundation of my second life. It wasn't glamorous. It wasn't always easy. But it was powerful. I realised that the most important decisions are the small ones we make every day. That's where transformation happens. Not in the loud, dramatic moments, but in the quiet, consistent ones.

You don't need to be perfect. You just need to show up, again and again.

Chapter 7

Movement is Medicine

There's a powerful truth I discovered during my healing journey: movement heals in ways medicine cannot. After my stroke, I wasn't just facing physical recovery, I was confronting fear, vulnerability, and disconnection from my own body. Movement became more than rehabilitation. It became my therapy, my way back to strength, and my declaration that I was not giving up.

I didn't need to become an athlete or chase extreme fitness goals. What I needed was to show up with gentleness, consistency, and intention. Slowly, one step at a time, I began to move again. And as I moved, something inside me shifted, not just physically, but emotionally and mentally. I wasn't just surviving anymore. I was beginning to thrive.

The Impact of Regular Movement on Mood, Heart, and Focus

In the early days, even a short walk lifted the heavy fog from my mind. A brisk 20-minute stroll gave me clarity, a boost of optimism, and a renewed sense of energy. That wasn't wishful thinking, it was biology in action. Regular movement improves blood flow, strengthens the heart, and activates powerful neurochemicals like dopamine, serotonin, and endorphins. These are your natural mood elevators, essential for motivation, emotional balance, and focus. According to

Healthdirect (n.d.), exercise not only supports physical wellbeing but also significantly boosts mental health by relieving symptoms of stress, anxiety, and depression.

After a neurological event like a stroke, these benefits aren't just helpful, they're vital. For me, movement became daily medicine. My sleep improved. My heart rate steadied. My thinking became clearer. I wasn't doing this for aesthetic gains, I was moving to heal. That shift in purpose changed everything. It wasn't optional. It was essential.

Simple, Sustainable Workouts, Walking, Gym, and Gentle Yoga

I didn't rush into intense workouts. I began where I was: with breath, intention, and gentle motion. At first, that meant slow walking, stretching, and basic posture awareness. As I gained strength, I gradually expanded my routine, always listening to my body, never pushing into pain or burnout.

Once my stroke consultant gave me the green light to return to the gym, I worked with a friend and trainer who understood my limitations and goals. Together, we created a plan that was both sustainable and empowering.

Here's what my movement routine looked like:

- *Walking***:** Every day, I walked at least 4–5 kilometres. It became a moving meditation—a time to think, breathe, and reconnect with nature.
- *Strength training (Gym):* Two to three times a week, I focused on building upper-body strength, chest, back, and shoulders. This not only improved my posture but also gave me confidence as a man rebuilding his physical presence.
- *Treadmill and light cardio:* 20–30-minute sessions supported my cardiovascular health and stamina.
- *Stretching and Yoga:* On off days, I practised gentle movements to maintain flexibility and reduce stress. This helped me avoid stiffness, especially during the colder UK months.

It wasn't about perfection. It was about presence, showing up for myself every day with care and commitment.

Seeing Progress, and Feeling Proud Again

Perhaps one of the most beautiful parts of this journey was seeing and feeling the change, not just in my body, but in my spirit.

As my stamina returned and my posture improved, I began to feel *in control again*. I could walk further, stand taller, and move with intention. These wins, small at first, turned into powerful milestones.

And with them came a deep, internal pride. Not the loud kind, but the quiet kind that says, "I'm showing up for myself." After the stroke, I felt like my body had failed me. But through consistent movement, I began to trust it again.

My clothes fit better. My energy stayed stable throughout the day. And more importantly, I felt *capable,* physically and emotionally. Friends and family noticed, not just in how I looked, but in how I carried myself.

Rebuilding Confidence Through the Body

Confidence isn't just a mindset; it's an embodied experience. When we feel strong, capable, and physically connected to ourselves, that radiates through every part of our lives.

For me, movement didn't just rebuild muscles, it rebuilt self-belief. Each stretch, each step, each drop of sweat whispered the same message: You're not broken. You're powerful. You're healing.

This physical consistency helped me rediscover trust in my body, and that trust gave me the courage to dream bigger, show up for my family, and lead with purpose.

Movement Is Your Medicine

Movement is not just a tool for recovery. It is a statement of self-respect. A form of gratitude. A silent but powerful affirmation: I am alive, and I am taking care of this body that carries me through life.

You don't need to run marathons. You don't need to lift heavy weights. You just need to move consistently, gently, and with love.

Walk. Stretch. Breathe. Dance. Move in ways that feel nourishing, not punishing. Your body will respond. Your spirit will rise.

Let your movement become your message:
I'm not just surviving, I'm thriving.

Chapter 8

Health is the First Wealth

There's a saying we've all heard: "Health is wealth." But how often do we truly live by it? Most of us keep it in the background, nodding at the wisdom of it, while continuing to push our bodies and minds to the limit, chasing career milestones, material goals, and social expectations. I know I did.

That is, until everything stopped.

When I suffered my stroke, the truth of that phrase hit me like a lightning bolt. My health had been trying to get my attention for years, through fatigue, poor sleep, high work pressure, and stress. But I ignored the signals. I believed I was too busy to slow down. Too successful to fall apart.

But the body keeps the score.

And that moment changed everything.

Suddenly, qualifications, career achievements, and the size of my bank account seemed meaningless; even though I could physically get up and move around, I was doing it without medical permission, against advice. I wasn't completely bedridden, but I felt the weight of vulnerability, the uncertainty that comes after a stroke. In that stripped-down moment, I wasn't measuring life by external success anymore. I realised something much deeper: Health is not just wealth; it is the very currency of life itself. Without it, nothing else holds real value.

Waking Up Without Pain: The Real Luxury

We live in a world that defines luxury through possessions, cars, watches, designer clothes, and houses. But none of those things compares to the luxury of waking up pain-free.

When half of your body goes numb and your speech slurs without warning, you stop seeing health as just another checkbox. You start to see it as sacred. Today, the ability to wake up, stretch both arms, feel both feet on the floor, and take a deep breath without discomfort, that's my new definition of abundance.

You don't think about these things when they're working. But once they're gone, you'll give anything to have them back. That's why I say now, with deep conviction: a peaceful body and a clear mind are the finest luxuries anyone can own.

No Career or Bank Balance Can Replace a Healthy Body

In the months following my stroke, I met many people, some patients, some caregivers, who shared the same regret: "I wish I had taken my health more seriously."

We often sacrifice our bodies at the altar of ambition. We skip meals, trade sleep for late-night work, ignore stress, and tell ourselves we'll rest later. But "later" is not promised, and for many, "later" becomes a hospital room, a diagnosis, or a permanent limitation.

Let me ask you something I asked myself in the mirror:

What use is your career title, your savings account, or your next promotion… if you're too sick to enjoy it?

We must stop treating health as an afterthought. It's not a reward for success; it's the foundation of it. Without your body functioning at its best, all your goals become harder to reach, and none of your achievements can be fully enjoyed.

Invest in Yourself First

Think of your health like a high-yield investment. The returns are incredible if you start now.

When you eat nourishing food, move daily, rest deeply, and protect your mental peace, you are making deposits into your health bank. And these deposits pay off, not just in longevity, but in the energy, clarity, and vitality you need to chase every dream.

Here's what I started doing, and what I still do today:

- I eat with intention, choosing foods that fuel my brain and calm inflammation.
- I move my body every single day, whether it's walking, strength training, or stretching.
- I prioritise sleep like my life depends on it, because it does.
- I say no to stress and yes to peace. That includes setting boundaries, meditating, and journaling.

And most importantly, I stopped seeing these as chores. I now see them as powerful, life-protecting rituals.

Remember: you can't pour from an empty cup. If you want to be there for your family, build your dreams, or make a lasting impact, you must invest in your well-being first.

A Life Lesson You Can Act on Today

You don't need to wait for a wake-up call like a stroke to start taking your health seriously. Prevention is the most powerful medicine.

So act today, even if it's small.

- Start your day with a glass of warm water.
- Go for a walk in nature.
- Eat one more vegetable and one less processed snack.

- Turn off your screens 30 minutes earlier and give your brain a break.
- Speak kindly to yourself. That's health, too.

You don't need a complete overhaul overnight. You just need to start.

Each small action creates momentum. And that momentum leads to transformation.

Final Thought

In the end, everything I've written in this chapter can be distilled into one truth:

Health isn't a side goal; it's the goal that supports all the others.

When you take care of your health, you're not just preventing illness. You're protecting your ability to love, to lead, to laugh, to create, and to live fully.

So, take it from someone who had to learn the hard way:
- The real bank account is your body.
- The real profit is peace of mind.
- And the richest life is a healthy life.

Chapter 9

Purpose, Not Pressure

There was a time in my life when every day felt like a race against the clock. I was always trying to do more, be more, and prove more. From the outside, it may have looked like ambition, but inside, I was living with a quiet storm of pressure. Expectations, whether from society, family, or myself, kept pushing me harder. And I kept going, believing that pressure was the fuel I needed to succeed.

Then came the stroke.

That one moment brought everything to a halt. The constant forward rush turned into stillness. The deadlines disappeared. All that remained was the question: What truly matters now?

That moment changed me. I stopped chasing and started reflecting. I didn't want to keep running, I wanted to walk with meaning. I didn't want to be driven by pressure, I wanted to be guided by purpose.

From Survival Mode to Meaningful Living

Before the stroke, life moved fast. I was focused on goals, responsibilities, and keeping things running. I didn't always take the time to pause or reflect, not because I didn't care, but because it felt like there was always something that needed to be done. Rest felt like something I had to earn, not something I naturally allowed. Even with achievements, there were moments when I felt something was missing. Looking back, I can see that I wasn't fully connected to myself; I was doing a lot, but not always being present.

After the stroke, I had to slow down, not just physically, but mentally and emotionally. And in that space, I found clarity.

Pressure depletes. Purpose renews.

Now, instead of asking, What's next? I ask, why now? I no longer take on tasks out of obligation or to maintain appearances. I choose what aligns with my values. I let go of the need to impress and instead focus on what truly inspires me.

This shift has given me more peace, more focus, and more fulfilment than I ever had during the busiest times of my life.

Reframing Goals: From Achievement to Alignment

I still set goals. I still believe in discipline, hard work, and progress. But now, my goals come from a different place. They aren't about proving myself or ticking boxes. They are about aligning my actions with my values and intentions.

For example:

- I'm writing this book not for recognition, but to share a message of hope and resilience with others.
- I manage my responsibilities not just to stay busy, but to stay connected to what matters most.
- I continue learning and growing, not to compete, but to stay curious, capable, and inspired.

This realignment has transformed how I live and work. It's no longer about arriving somewhere. It's about walking the right path, even if it's slower.

Living More Meaningfully, One Day at a Time

Living with purpose doesn't require a complete life overhaul. It begins with small, consistent decisions:

- Choosing rest over overcommitment.
- Saying no to things that drain you, even if they seem "important."
- Spending time with people who lift you.
- Starting each morning with gratitude for being alive.

Since the stroke, I've simplified many things. I no longer fill my calendar to feel worthy. I don't say yes out of guilt. I listen to my body, honour my energy, and focus on what nourishes me.

That doesn't mean I've stopped growing. It means I've started growing in the right direction.

Guided by Values, Not Just Urgency

I've learned to live by a few guiding values:
- **Health over hustle**
- **Purpose over pressure**
- **Presence over perfection**
- **Meaning over metrics**

These values act like a compass. When I feel overwhelmed or lost, I return to them. They bring me back to what matters.

And here's the surprising truth: living this way hasn't made me less effective. It's made me more focused. My relationships are deeper. My decisions are clearer. My sense of self is stronger.

Because when you live with purpose, even the smallest steps move you forward.

Final Reflection

Letting go of pressure doesn't mean letting go of ambition. It means choosing a healthier, more sustainable way to grow.

I used to believe pressure was necessary to achieve. But now I know that purpose is more powerful. It doesn't burn you out, it builds you up.

So, here's my message to you:

You don't have to chase everything.

You don't have to prove anything.

You just need to live intentionally, with heart, with honesty, and with purpose.

Because when you live with purpose, you don't just survive, you thrive.

Chapter 10

My New Beginning

This chapter isn't the end of my story.
It's the beginning of the rest of my life.

When I look back at that moment, the stroke that shook my world, it no longer feels like a tragedy. It was a turning point. A hard reset. A sacred invitation to live differently.

I didn't just recover. I was reborn.

A Celebration of My Second Chance

Waking up after the stroke was one of the most terrifying experiences of my life. My body didn't feel like mine. My mind was clouded. My future was uncertain.

But today, I wake up with energy, clarity, and purpose. I see life differently. I celebrate small things, quiet mornings, my son's laughter, a peaceful walk, and a full breath. I don't take any of it for granted.

This second chance isn't just about physical healing. It's about becoming the version of myself I was always meant to be.

Yes, I've changed my lifestyle. Yes, I've transformed my habits.
But more than that, I've changed my identity.

This Wasn't the End, It Was the Rebirth

So many people think illness is the end of the road. But often, it's just the beginning of a better path. My stroke felt like a full stop, but it turned out to be a comma. A pause. A shift.

Before, I was running too fast to notice what I was missing. Now, I walk with intention. I see more. I feel more. I am more.

That's why I call this my new beginning.
Not because I've forgotten the past, but because I've learned from it.
Not because I returned to my old self, but because I created someone new.

This experience didn't just change me. It elevated me.

I Am Not Just a Survivor, I Am a Life Transformer

It's easy to wear the badge of "survivor." But I want more than survival. I want *transformation*. I didn't go through all this just to go back to where I was. I went through it to evolve.

Now I'm not just living, I'm *leading*. I'm teaching others what I've learned. I'm using my story, my mistakes, and my recovery as tools to inspire healing in others.

I've become a better father. A wiser husband. A more grounded friend.

A more present human being.

And the most powerful thing is, I *chose* this path.

I didn't stay stuck in pain, or fear, or regret. I accepted my story, then rewrote the ending.

And if I can do that, so can you.

Your Invitation to Begin Again

Maybe you haven't had a stroke. Maybe your pain is invisible. Maybe your burnout is quiet. Maybe you've been drifting, waiting for a wake-up call that hasn't come yet.

Let this chapter be your call.

You don't need a medical crisis to start over. You don't need to wait for rock bottom to climb upward. You don't need anyone's permission to rewrite your story.

You can begin again today. Right now.

Start with one better decision. One small shift. One commitment to take back control of your health, your mind, your habits, and your energy.

You are not broken. You are rebuilding.
You are not stuck. You are realigning.
You are not late. You are right on time.

Final Words

This book began with a moment that nearly ended my life.

It ends with the moment I claimed it back.

From patient to power. From breakdown to breakthrough.

From fear to faith. From surviving to transforming.

This is my new beginning.

And I hope, with all my heart, it becomes the start of *yours* too.

Let's walk forward together, stronger, wiser, and more alive than ever.

References

American Stroke Association. (2025). *Transient ischemic attack (TIA)*. https://www.stroke.org/en/about-stroke/types-of-stroke/tia-transient-ischemic-attack

Chaput, J.-P., Després, J.-P., Bouchard, C., & Tremblay, A. (2014). Sleep patterns, diet quality, and lipid profile in the Quebec Family Study. *The American Journal of Clinical Nutrition, 79*(4), 630–636. https://doi.org/10.1093/ajcn/79.4.630

Healthdirect. (n.d.). *Exercise and mental health*. Healthdirect Australia. https://www.healthdirect.gov.au/exercise-and-mental-health

Horne, J. A., & Pankhurst, F. (2017). Late-night eating and its effects on metabolic health: A review of the evidence. *The Journal of Sleep Research, 26*(3), 280–285. https://doi.org/10.1111/jsr.12382

Kris-Etherton, P. M., Petersen, K. S., Hibbeln, J. R., Hurley, D., Kolick, V., Peoples, S., Rodriguez, N. R., & Thomas, R. J. (2021). Nutrition and behavioral health disorders: Depression and anxiety. *Nutrition Reviews, 79*(3), 247–260. https://doi.org/10.1093/nutrit/nuaa025

Lustig, R. H., Schmidt, L. A., & Brindis, C. D. (2012). The toxic truth about sugar. *Nature, 482*(7383), 27–29. https://doi.org/10.1038/482027a

Manohar, P. R., Eranezhath, S., Mahapatra, A., & Manohar, S. R. (2021). Panchakarma therapies: An overview of the evidence and modern relevance. *Journal of Ayurveda and Integrative Medicine, 12*(3), 420–427. https://doi.org/10.1016/j.jaim.2020.07.006

Mayo Clinic. (2024). *Transient ischemic attack (TIA)*. https://www.mayoclinic.org/diseases-conditions/transient-ischemic-attack/symptoms-causes/syc-20355679

Patwardhan, B., Warude, D., Pushpangadan, P., & Bhatt, N. (2005). Ayurveda and traditional Chinese medicine: A comparative overview. *Evidence-Based Complementary and Alternative Medicine, 2*(4), 465–473. https://doi.org/10.1093/ecam/neh140

Walker, M. (2017). *Why we sleep: Unlocking the power of sleep and dreams*. Scribner.

World Health Organization (WHO). (2023). *Obesity and overweight*. https://www.who.int/news-room/fact-sheets/detail/obesity-and-overweight

World Obesity Federation. (2024). *World Obesity Atlas 2024*. https://www.worldobesity.org/resources/resource-library/world-obesity-atlas-2024

Zeevi, D., Korem, T., Zmora, N., Israeli, D., Rothschild, D., Weinberger, A., ... & Segal, E. (2015). Personalized nutrition by prediction of glycemic responses. *Cell, 163*(5), 1079–1094. https://doi.org/10.1016/j.cell.2015.11.001

About the Author

Channa A. G. is a UK-based professional with a diverse background in Ayurveda, international business, artificial intelligence, and politics.

He holds a degree in Ayurvedic Medicine and Surgery from the University of Colombo, Sri Lanka, a master's in international business management from Northumbria University in the UK, and a certification in Artificial Intelligence from the University of Oxford. He is also planning to begin a BA in British Politics and Legislative Studies at the University of Hull in the 2025/26 academic year.

As an entrepreneur, Channa has built and led multiple successful ventures across a range of industries. His strategic mindset, combined with a deep respect for both tradition and innovation, shapes his work and worldview.

Now living in the UK, Channa devotes his time to writing, business development, and personal transformation. *From Patient to Power* is not just a record of recovery, it's a reflection of his belief that setbacks can become turning points, and that healing is the beginning of something greater.

Other Books by the Author

Small Steps to Smart Business
A Practical Guide for New Entrepreneurs

In this practical and encouraging guide, Channa A. G. shares essential tools, mindset shifts, and real-world strategies to help aspiring entrepreneurs take confident steps toward building successful businesses. Whether you're just starting or refining your vision, this book offers clear, actionable advice to turn small beginnings into smart growth.

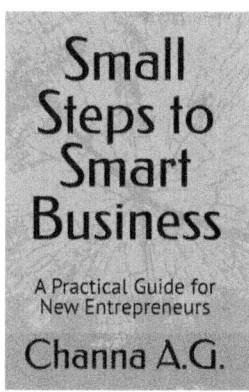

Small Steps to Smart Business
A Practical Guide for New Entrepreneurs
Now available on Amazon.

▪ Scan the QR code below to get your copy!

Stay Connected

Thank you for reading *From Patient to Power*.

I hope it offered insight, inspiration, and encouragement for your own journey. My path continues to evolve, and I'd love to stay connected with you as I explore healing, business, AI, and purposeful living.

You can follow my work and reflections here:

Website: www.dachayurveda.com
Email: channaaguk@gmail.com
Facebook: facebook.com/drchannajinasena
Instagram: instagram.com/channa_a_g
X (Twitter): twitter.com/Channa_AG
LinkedIn: linkedin.com/in/channa-a-g

If this book resonated with you, please consider leaving a review on Amazon. Your feedback helps others discover it, and it truly means a lot to me.

Let's keep the conversation going.

Printed in Great Britain
by Amazon